Sirtfood Diet Guidebook

A Straightforward Guide To Master The Art Of An Amazing Diet That Helps You Lose Weight In 1 Week

Zelda Hum

© Copyright 2021 - All rights reserved.

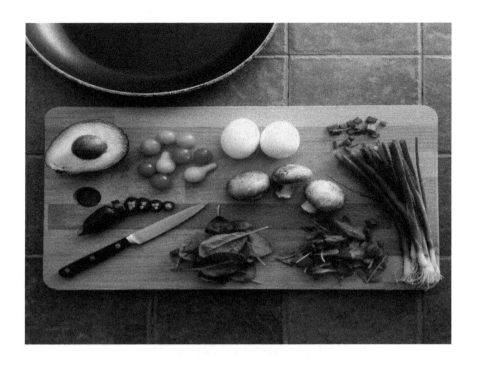

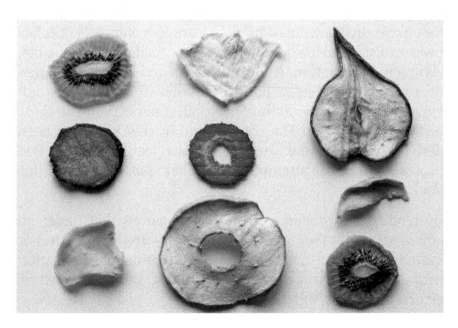

Table of Contents

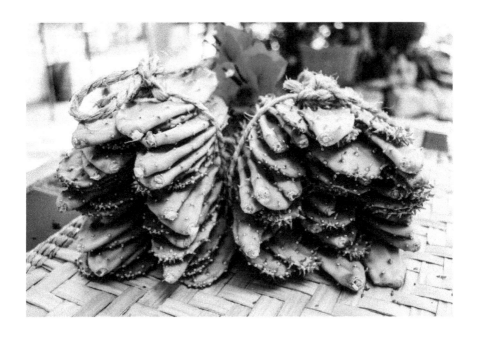

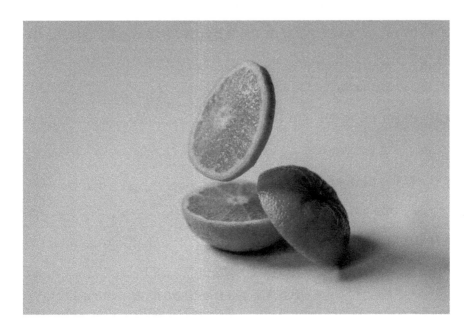

INTRODUCTION:

As explained by the diet administrators, these particular nourishments act by initiating simple proteins in the body called sirtuins. Sirtuins are approved to protect the cells of the body from dying when under stress and are expected to regulate agitation, metabolism, and the process of aging. It is the assumption that sirtuins hinder the capacity of the body to consume fat and lift digestion, resulting in seven-pound weight loss after taking care of muscle for seven days. A few researchers, however, believe that this is not likely to be a strictly fat reduction but also would reflect changes in the stocks of muscle tissue and liver glycogen.

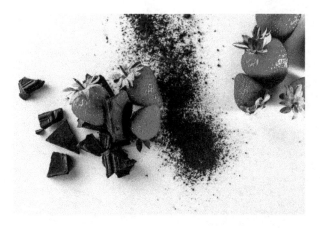

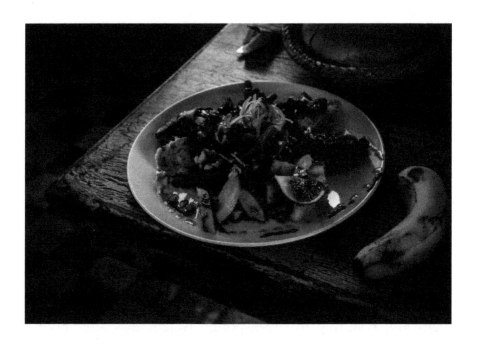

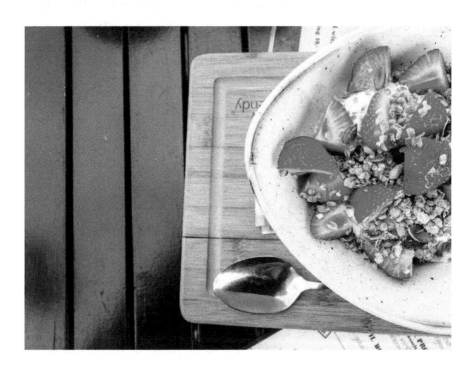

CHAPTER 1:
What is the Sirtfood Diet?

This chapter will help you understand the importance of the Sirtfood Diet. In the United Kingdom, two celebrity nutritionists collaborating with a health club founded The Sirtfood Diet. They market the diet as a groundbreaking modern health and wellbeing strategy that works by turning on the "skinny gene," This diet focuses on Sirtuin (SIRT) research, a group of seven body proteins that have been shown to regulate numerous roles, inflammation, including metabolism and lifespan. Certain organic plant compounds can increase the number of such proteins, and diets containing them have been called 'Sirt foods.'

The Sirtfood Diet's listing of the "Top 20 Sirtfoods" includes:

- Extra-virgin Olive Oil

- Dark Chocolate (85% Cocoa)

- Matcha Green Tea

- Buckwheat

- Turmeric

- Walnuts

- Arugula (Rocket)

- Bird's Eye Chili

- Lovage

- Kale

- Red Wine

- Strawberries

- Onions

- Soy

- Parsley

- Medjool Dates

- Red Chicory

- Blueberries

- Capers

- Coffee

In the diet, Sirtfoods and calorie restriction are mixed, enabling the body to produce greater amounts of Sirtuins. The diet creators suggest it will result in dramatic weight loss by following the Sirtfood Diet while maintaining muscle mass and protecting you from chronic disease. After completing the diet, all are allowed to start adding sirtfoods and the diet's signature green juice into their regular diet

1.1. After the Diet

For more weight loss, you can repeat these subsequent steps as much as you can.

Nevertheless, you are encouraged to practice "sirtifying" the diet after finishing these stages by integrating sirtfoods every day through your meals.

On Sirtfood Diet, there is a lot of literature full of sirtfood-rich recipes. It is also possible to use Sirtfoods in dishes or as a snack you already have in your diet.

You are also advised to try to eat green juice each day.

In this manner, Sirtfood Diet seems to be more of a routine transformation than a single-time diet.

1.2. Sirtfoods as Superfoods

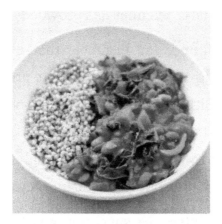

There is no doubt that at sirtfoods, you are amazing. Nutrients & full safe Earth goods are also abundant in them.

Also, the study has related beneficial effects to various of the products suggested on Sirtfood Diet.

For starters, eating moderate doses of the dark chocolate along with such a high quantity cocoa content will decrease the danger of heart problems and help battle inflammation.

Consuming green tea will decrease the rate of strokes and diabetes & help reduce blood pressure.And the turmeric has anti-inflammatory characteristics, typically having advantageous effects on body and defending against inflammation-related chronic diseases.

In human beings, the bulk of Sirt foods have confirmed health benefits.

However, preliminary reports are available on health effects of increasing quantities of a protein from Sirtuin. Even the research of animals & cell lines has provided exciting results.

Observers also found, for instance, that elevated levels in worms, yeast, and mice of some sirtuin protein result to a longer lifespan. Sirtuin proteins warn the body during calorie restriction or fasting to burn additional fat for the energy & increase sensitivity of insulin. One analysis in mice has demonstrated that higher levels of Sirtuin contribute to lose fat.

Both pieces of the literature suggest that sirtuins can also help suppress inflammation, prevent tumor growth, and slows the growth of Alzheimer's and high cholesterol. While experiments have shown positive results in human and mice cell lines, the effects of increased levels of Sirtuin have not been studied in human studies. If elevated levels of sirtuin protein in body lead to a extended lifespan or a lesser incidence of human cancer is still uncertain.

Research is presently underway to produce compounds that are successful at raising amounts of Sirtuin in body. This method, the human research will start to investigate the influence of sirtuins on human wellbeing.

The results of elevated levels of a sirtuin will not be identified by then.

1.3. Sirtfoods is Balanced and Sustainable

Sirtfoods are nearly always safe choices and can, due to the anti-inflammatory or antioxidant properties, even result in beneficial effects.

Yet, eating only a a few of predominantly healthy foods does not meet all the body's dietary needs.

Sirtfood Diet is overly restrictive and does not give any other diet any basic, special beneficial effects.

Also, under a doctor's supervision, it is naturally not suggested to eat just 1,000 calories. For certain persons, also consuming 1,500 calories a day is overly restricting.

Eating up to 3 green juices a day is also included in the diet. Even though the juices consider to be a decent provider of vitamins, they are as well the source of sugars & hardly contain any nutritional fiber carried by whole vegetables and fruits.

What's worse, drinking juice all day is not good thing both for your teeth and your blood sugar.

Not to refer, as diet is so restricted in food choices and calories, proteins, vitamins and minerals are more than probable to be insufficient, especially in the first step.

The daily suggested quantity of protein, for example, varies between 2 & 6.5 pounds equivalents & depends on many factors, including many variables:

- **How old are you.**

- **Whether you are female or male.**

- **How active are you.**

This diet can be tough to manage for 3-weeks due to low-calorie levels and minimal food choices.

Add to it the high early expense of having a juicer, a journal and some rare and unusual ingredients, and the time cost of preparing various foods and drinks, and for most people, this diet turns out to be extremely expensive pricey and impractical.

1.4. Protections and side-effects

While the first step of Sirtfood Diet is quite low in the calories & nutritionally inadequate, given the diet's limited duration, there are no clear safety risks for the typical healthy adult.

However, calorie constraint & only juice intake for initial few days of a diet for those with diabetes will cause unsafe changes in the blood sugar level.

Even a stable person, after all, will experience such adverse effects, mostly hunger.

Trying to eat only the 1,000 to 1,500 calories a day shall leave just around any one feeling hungry, especially if low-fat juice, a nutrient which helps to keep you sensing full, is a lot of what you drink.

You will experience additional side-effects all over phase one, such as lightheadedness, irritability, and fatigue due to dietary changes.

For an otherwise healthy patient, serious health penalties are improbable if diet is observed only for Three weeks.

1.5. From the Bottom Line

Nutritious foods, but not healthy eating habits, are packed with Sirtfood Diet.

It is not to refer that it is based on broad extrapolations of its theories and health arguments from preliminary science evidence.

However, accumulating some of the Sirtfoods to diet isn't bad and may also have some health benefits; diet itself seems to be just another trend.

Save your own money and failing to make healthy long-term lifestyle improvements.

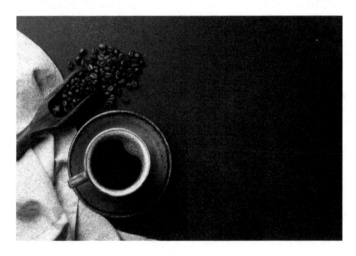

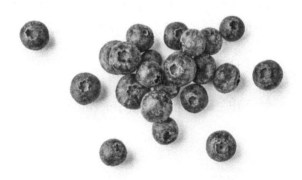

CHAPTER 2:
The 21-day Sirtfood Diet Plan

Think chapter is devoted to the diet plan of sirtfood that I attempted personally and on which I could lose weight in the long term without the yo-yo impact. I want to announce that as a warning, the first few days are pretty. After that, especially if you want to cook and serve, the plan is very fun and pretty simple to execute. The rest of the time works by itself as soon as you have made it past the first three days. I want to mention that if you do not manage to adhere to the diet the first time, there is no guilt. Trying two, three or four times and then working is better than trying none at all. A little advice from me to eliminate all food unsuitable for the diet and all the little vices of daily life from your house or apartment is necessary for the period before the 21 days. You don't want to make the first three days more complicated, after all than they are now. After completing each process, I would also suggest that you maintain a log of how you felt. It helps a lot to be able to show your anger during the diet! You can stretch stage 2 as long as you want until you have achieved the target weight. The turn back to a larger calorie requirement, i.e., regular eating behavior, is step 3. It is important to sustain the eating rhythm, the calorie requirement and the consistency in the diet after phase 3 to stay lower in the long term. Nevertheless, you no longer need to be based on sirtfoods. If you follow a different, balanced diet, it is not a concern. I warmly and desperately suggest some fitness and sport at the same time! So, you don't have to go to a sports class, a climbing club or a gym every day like I do, but it's very good to do some daily workout or running three or four days a week, not only to lose weight but also for your bones and joints and your cycle. It is possible to replicate the strategy many times, too. That means you can go through it once, take a couple of weeks off, and then go through the diet again. Let's not waste more words, however, and begin with the plan!

2.1. Phase 1. 1000 kcal per day

Day 1.

1.Smoothie: Original Sirtfood Smoothie (300 kcal)

Main meal: spinach nests + 1 slice of superfood bread (350 kcal)

2. Smoothie: Green Juice (300 kcal)

Day 2.

1.Smoothie: Cucumber Smoothie (300 kcal)

 Main meal: mushroom-spinach omelet + 1 slice of superfood bread (450 kcal)

3.Smoothie: Green smoothie with mint (300 kcal)

Day 3.

1.Smoothie: Celery Smoothie (300 kcal)

Main meal: Zucchini noodles with tofu (350 kcal)

3.Smoothie: Original Sirtfood Smoothie (300 kcal)

2.2. Phase 2. 1500 kcal per day

Day 4.

Breakfast: yogurt parfait with berries (350 kcal)

Lunch: A smoothie of your choice (300 kcal)

Snack: Mango Nice-Cream (400 kcal)

Dinner: Stuffed avocado with chicken + 1 slice of superfood bread (400 kcal)

Day 5.

Breakfast: low-carbohydrate pancakes (252 kcal) + topping of your choice (50-100 kcal)

Lunch: 2 eggs in a glass with 2-slices of superfood bread (500 kcal)

Snack: papaya carpaccio (11.0 kcal) + 2 apples with peanut butter (120 kcal)

Dinner: A smoothie of your choice (300 kcal)

Day 6.

Breakfast: Banana Chocolate Cream (350 kcal)

Lunch: A smoothie of your choice (300 kcal)

Snack: blueberry nice cream (350 kcal)

Dinner: Waldorf Salad (450 kcal)

Day 7.

Breakfast: spinach nests + 2 slices of superfood bread (450 kcal)

Lunch: grapefruit-avocado salad with 1-slice of superfood bread (500 kcal)

Snack: vegetable sticks with guacamole (250 kcal)

Dinner: A smoothie of your choice (300 kcal)

Day 8.

Breakfast: Avocado Eggs with Salsa Dip (480 kcal)

Lunch: A smoothie of your choice (300 kcal)

Snack: Vanilla yogurt (180 kcal)

Dinner: Cauliflower Pizza with Smoked Salmon (600 kcal)

Day 9.

Breakfast: Chia pudding with blueberries and banana (250 kcal)

Lunch: Buckwheat Bowl (400)

Snack: Finger food plate: 6 large black olives, 50g pomegranate seeds, a handful of berries (175 kcal)

Dinner: A smoothie of your choice in double portion or two different smoothies (600 kcal)

Day 10.

Breakfast: pineapple yogurt with banana and peanuts (300 kcal)

Lunch: A smoothie of your choice in double portions or two different smoothies (600 kcal)

Snack: Vegetable sticks with salsa dip (150 kcal)

Dinner: Egg-Broccoli Salad (360 kcal)

Day 11.

Breakfast: Quinoa breakfast (421 kcal)

Lunch: Stuffed peppers with spinach and egg + two slices of superfood bread (450 kcal)

Snack: 10 grapes (30 kcal)

Dinner: A smoothie of your choice in double portion or two different smoothies (600 kcal)

Day 12.

Breakfast: Avocado Eggs with Salsa Dip (480 kcal)

Lunch: A smoothie of your choice (300 kcal)

Snack: soy milkshake (138 kcal)

Dinner: Cauliflower Salad (560 kcal)

Day 13.

Breakfast: low-carbohydrate pancakes (252 kcal) with the topping of your choice (100

kcal)

Lunch: A smoothie of your choice (300 kcal)

Snack: Berries Nice Cream (300 kcal)

Dinner: kale soup (560 kcal)

Day 14.

Breakfast: porridge made from coconut flour with the topping of your choice (350 kcal)

Lunch: stuffed peppers with spinach you. Egg (200 kcal)

Snack: low carb waffles with 2-apples and peanut butter (300 kcal)

Dinner: A smoothie of your choice in double serving or two different smoothies (600 kcal)

2.3. Phase 3. 1800 kcal per day

Day 15.

Breakfast: Avocado Eggs with Salsa Dip (480)

Lunch: Vegan noodle pan (550)

Snack: Apple carpaccio with spring quark (350)

Dinner: Bean Stew (500)

Day 16.

Breakfast: Quinoa breakfast (421 kcal)

Lunch: Asian noodle pan with tofu (550 kcal)

Snack: Crostini with tapenade (400 kcal)

Dinner: Quinoa with vegetables (470 kcal)

Day 17.

Breakfast: cottage cheese crunch (490 kcal)

Lunch: Eggplant Wedges with Pesto (500 kcal)

Snack: Colorful salad (300 kcal)

Dinner: Whole grain pita (500 kcal)

Day 18.

Breakfast: bread with egg and avocado (415 kcal)

Lunch: Sirt Super Salad (450 kcal)

Snack: Shakshuka (250 kcal)

Dinner: Sirtfood Pizza (600 kcal)

Day 19.

Breakfast: Mango Nice Cream (400 kcal)

Lunch: Braised Lentils (500 kcal)

Snack: 4 Energy Bites (350 kcal)

Dinner: Potato and kale soup (560 kcal)

Day 20:

Breakfast: Chia yogurt with clementine puree (450 kcal)

Lunch: kidney beans with baked potatoes (450 kcal)

Snack: Blueberry Nice Cream (400 kcal)

Dinner: Butternut Tajine (550 kcal)

Day 21.

Breakfast: Avocado Eggs with Salsa Dip (480 kcal)

Lunch: Fruity pasta salad (570 kcal)

Snack: 4 Energy Bites (350 kcal)

Dinner: Harissa Tofu with Cauliflower Couscous (450 kcal)

CHAPTER 3:

Breakfast Recipes

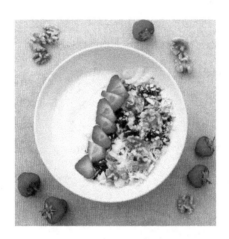

The step-by-step method of making delicious, mouth-watering sirtfood dishes that are great for breakfast will be investigated. These ingredients were specifically chosen to provide you with the stamina and vigor you will need to do well during the day while helping you stay balanced, lose unhealthy weight and look great. Let's dive in!

1. Savory Buckwheat Bowls

(Serving: 2, Cooking time: 30 minutes, Difficulty: Normal)

Ingredients:

- Buckwheat groats, toasted – 1 cup

- Extra virgin olive oil – 1 tablespoon

- Water – 2 cups

- Sea salt - .25 teaspoon

- Onion, diced – .5

- Button mushrooms, sliced – 4

- Parsley, chopped – 2 tablespoons

- Eggs – 2

- Capers, drained – 1 tablespoon

Instructions:

1. Rinse and transfer the buckwheat along with the water and sea salt to a saucepan. Over medium heat, cook the buckwheat groats until the water has been absorbed and the groats are fluffy. Remove from the sun, cover with a lid, and sit for 10 minutes with the groats.

2. Meanwhile, add to the pan the extra virgin olive oil and onion, along with a tiny sprinkle of sea salt. Enable the onion to cook slowly over low heat until the caramelized onion is darkened, stirring regularly. Bring in the parsley and mushrooms and saute for five minutes until the mushrooms are tender.

3. In the skillet, add the cooked buckwheat, mix it and encourage the flavors to meld and cook together for an additional two minutes.

4. When your buckwheat finishes frying, prepare your eggs in a separate pan according to your choice. Cover the cooked eggs and capers with the buckwheat, then serve immediately.

2. Sweet Potato and Apple Breakfast Skillet

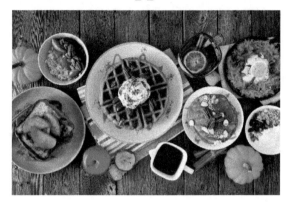

(Serving: 4, Cooking time: 30 minutes, Difficulty: Normal)

Ingredients:

- Extra virgin olive oil – 1 tablespoon

- Apple, diced – 1 Garlic, minced – 2 cloves

- Red onion, diced – 1 Sweet potato, peeled and diced – 1

- Black pepper, ground - .25 teaspoon

- Kale, chopped – 2 cups

- Chicken apple sausage, sliced – 4 links

- Sea salt - .5 teaspoon

Instructions:

1. In a big cast iron skillet, pour the olive oil and allow it to melt over medium heat. Connect the sweet potatoes and the onion and simmer for about seven minutes, until tender.

2. In the pan, add the sliced sausage and apple, allowing it to cook for an additional five minutes, making sure to stir regularly.

3. Stir in the seasonings and kale, allowing it to cook for a few more minutes, only before the kale is wilted. Take the sweet potato skillet off the fire and serve with eggs or alone.

3. Cinnamon Apple Quinoa

(Serving: 2, Cooking time: 25 minutes, Difficulty: Normal)

Ingredients:

- Quinoa - .5 cup

- Water – 1.5 cups

- Apples, peeled and diced – 2

- Cinnamon – 2 teaspoons

- Sea salt - .25 teaspoon

- Honey – 2 tablespoons

Instructions:

1. To a saucepan, add the apples, quinoa, sea salt and water. Before reducing the heat to a minimum, bring the water, apples, and quinoa to a boil and cover the quinoa mixture with a lid and enable it to simmer for around twenty minutes. It is ready when the quinoa has drained the water, and the apples are tender.

2. Stir in the cinnamon and split the quinoa into two dishes for eating. Drizzle over the top of the honey before loving.

4. Triple Berry Millet Bake

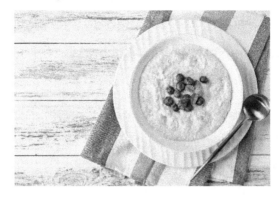

(Serving: 8, Cooking time: 70 minutes, Difficulty: Normal)

Ingredients:

- Millet – 1.5 cups

- Soy milk, unsweetened – 2 cups

- Water – 1 cup

- Date sugar - .5 cup

- Vanilla extract – 2 teaspoons

- Sea salt - .25 teaspoon

- Cinnamon - .5 teaspoon

- Walnuts, chopped – 1 cup

- Blueberries, thawed if frozen – 12 ounces

- Strawberries, sliced, thawed if frozen – 8 ounces

- Raspberries, thawed if frozen – 8 ounces

Instructions:

1. Set the oven to three hundred- and seventy-five-degrees Fahrenheit and prepare a 9-inch glass for a 13-inch baking dish.

2. Whisk the soy milk, water, millet, date sugar, cinnamon, sea salt, and vanilla extract together in a large kitchen dish. In the prepared pan, pour the mixture into it.

3. Sprinkle generously over the top of the plate with the berries and almonds, and then use a spatula or spoon to press the nuts back into the mixture gently.

4. Bake the millet for about one hour until it is hot and bubbling. Remove the millet from the oven and allow it to sit before serving for 15 minutes.

5. Green Shakshuka

(Serving: 3, Cooking time: 20 minutes, Difficulty: Normal)

Ingredients:

- Zucchini, grated – 1

- Brussels sprouts, finely sliced or shaved – 9 ounces

- Red onion, diced – 1

- Olive oil – 2 tablespoons

- Eggs – 5 Parsley, chopped - .25 cup

- Kale, chopped – 2 cups

- Sea salt - .5 teaspoon

- Cumin – 1 teaspoon

- Avocado, sliced – 1

Instructions:

1. Sauté the red onion in the olive oil in a wide steel skillet for about three minutes before it becomes partially translucent. Add in the minced garlic and cook the mixture of onion/garlic for an extra minute.

2. In the skillet containing the onion and garlic, add the Brussels sprouts and roast for four to five minutes until

softened, stirring regularly. Stir in the spices and zucchini, then simmer for an extra minute.

3. Stir in the skillet with the kale and continue stirring until it starts to wilt. Lower the heat to a low level.

4. The shakshuka mixture in the skillet is flattened with a spatula, and five small wells are formed for the eggs to come in. In each of the shakshuka wells, crack an egg and cover the skillet with a lid to steam the eggs until they fit your taste.

5. Round the dish off with the avocado and parsley, and serve immediately.

6. Kale and Butternut Bowls

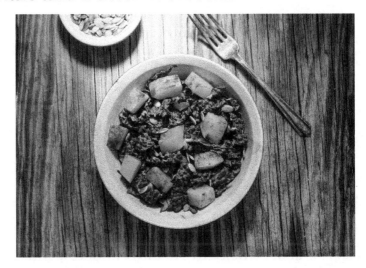

(Serving: 4, Cooking time: 60 Minutes, Difficulty: Normal)

Ingredients:

- Red onion, diced – 1

- Butternut squash, seeds removed and cut into quarters – 1

- Kale, chopped – 3 cups

- Garlic, minced – 2 cloves

- Extra virgin olive oil – 1 tablespoon

- Oregano, dried – 1 teaspoon

- Cinnamon - .25 teaspoon

- Turmeric powder - .5 teaspoon

- Sea salt – 1 teaspoon

- Avocado, sliced – 1 Eggs – 4

- Parsley, chopped - .25 cup

- Black pepper, ground - .25 teaspoon

Instructions:

1. Set the oven at four hundred- and twenty-degrees Fahrenheit. Place the butternut squash upside down on a pan so that the side of the skin faces upward. Roast the butternut squash for about twenty-five to thirty minutes, until the pork is tender.

2. Enable the butternut squash to cool down enough to be easy to touch, and then peel your hands off the flesh. Break the butternut squash into bite-size cubes.

3. Heat the extra virgin olive oil over a moderate medium - high heat skillet and sauté the onion for about five minutes until it is translucent. Connect the kale, garlic, and seasonings and simmer until the kale wilts. In the butternut squash, add.

4. Divide the skillet mixture into four serving bowls and finish each with your favorite fried egg, sliced avocado, and parsley.

7. Egg Casserole

(Serving: 6, Cooking time: 40 minutes, Difficulty: Normal)

Ingredients:

- Eggs – 10

- Breakfast sausage – 1 pound

- Button mushrooms, sliced – 2 cups

- Roma tomatoes, seeded and diced – 3

- Red onion, thinly sliced – 1

- Kale, chopped – 2 cups

- Basil, chopped – 1 tablespoon

- Parsley, chopped – 2 tablespoons

- Sea salt – 1.5 teaspoons

Instructions:

1. Set the oven to three hundred (300 degrees Fahrenheit) and prepare a thirteen-inch by nine-inch baking dish.

2. Your breakfast sausage, when thoroughly finished, draining off any extra fat in a skillet over medium-high brown.

3. Add the mushrooms to the skillet with the breakfast sausage, allowing them to saute for around five to seven minutes, until

tender. Add the remaining vegetables and sea salt and simmer for an additional two to three minutes until just slightly tender.

4. To the prepared pan, move the vegetable sausage mixture.

5. In a complete cup, whisk the eggs together, ensuring the whites thoroughly down into the yolks. For about twenty-five to thirty minutes, pour the eggs over the breakfast sausage, mix the vegetables, and then place it in the oven to roast until cooked through.

8. Vegan Tofu Omelette

(Serving: 1, Cooking time: 15 minutes, Difficulty: Easy)

Ingredients:

- Silken tofu – 6 ounces Tahini – 1 teaspoon (optional)

- Corn-starch – 1 tablespoon   Nutritional yeast – 1 tablespoon

- Soy milk, unsweetened – 1 tablespoon

- Turmeric, ground - .125 teaspoon Onion powder - .25 teaspoon

- Sea salt - .25 teaspoon Smoked paprika – .125 teaspoon (optional)

- Black salt - .25 teaspoon

- Kale, chopped - .5 cup Button mushrooms, sliced - .25 cup

- Onion, diced – 2 tablespoons

- Garlic, minced – 1 clove   Extra virgin olive oil – 1 tablespoon, dived

Instructions:

1. Add the tofu, tahini, maize starch, yeast, soy milk, turmeric, onion powder, smoked paprika, and all salts to a blender. Pulse on high until thoroughly mixed with the mixture.

2. Apply part of the olive oil along with the vegetables and garlic to a skillet. Saute until they are soft, over medium heat for around five minutes.

3. Meanwhile, over medium-high flame, pour the remaining half of the olive oil into a non-stick medium skillet. Enable this skillet to preheat until it is scalding when you are cooking the vegetables. When heated, apply the tofu batter to the skillet, tilting the pan slightly so that the egg forms a spherical shape. You should smooth out the surface with a spoon.

4. Sprinkle the cooked vegetables over the "egg" tofu and decrease the skillet heat to medium-low. Cover the skillet with a lid, allowing it to cook until the "egg" tofu is set and the sides have dried for three to five minutes. To gently raise the omelette's sides to ensure it is completely assembled, you can use a spatula. The shading, with few brown spots, should be golden.

5. Loosen the omelette by raising it with the spatula until it is ready, and then flip one side over the other. Switch the omelette of tofu to a plate and eat it when soft.

9. Vegetable Omelette

(Serving: 1, Cooking time: 15 minutes, Difficulty: Easy)

Ingredients:

- Eggs – 2 Extra virgin olive oil – 1 tablespoon, divided

- Soy milk, unsweetened – 1 teaspoon

- Sea salt - .5 teaspoon

- Lemon juice – 1 tablespoon

- Kale, chopped – 1 cup

- Parsley, chopped – 1 tablespoon

- Red pepper flakes - .125 teaspoon

- Avocado, sliced - .5

Instructions:

1. Whisk together the eggs, half the sea salt, and the soy milk in a tiny kitchen bowl until the eggs are moist and the yolk is entirely white.

2. Pour half of the olive oil into a medium pan, then cook over medium heat. Apply the lemon juice, part of the sea salt, and the red pepper flakes to the kale parsley. Cook for about three minutes, until the kale is soft and wilted. Out of the skillet, move the vegetables.

3. Pour the renamed olive oil into the hot saucepan and apply to the eggs. Please enable them to cook until it starts to set circularly, but the core is still slightly runny. It's going to take about three minutes.

4. To sandwich the vegetables between the two pieces, layer the cooked vegetables and sliced avocado over the egg and then flip one half of the egg over the other. Plate and serve the omelette when soft.

CHAPTER 4:

Main Dishes Recipes

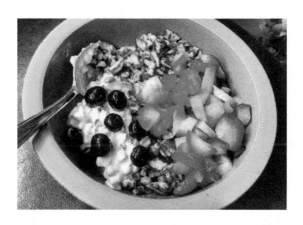

We'd discuss fabulous recipes of sirtfood that can preferably be made for lunch or dinner.

10.   Sirt super salad

(Serving: 1, Cooking time: 25 Minutes, Difficulty: Normal)

Ingredients:

- 1 3 / 4-ounce (50g) arugula

- 1 3 / 4-ounce (50g) endive leaves

- 3 1 / 2 ounces (100g) smoked salmon slices

- 1 / 2 cup (80g) avocado, peeled, stoned, and sliced

- 1 / 2 cup (50g) celery including leaves, sliced

- 1 / 8 cup (20g) red onion, sliced

- 1 / 8 cups (15g) walnuts, chopped

- 1 tablespoon capers

- 1 large Medjool date, pitted and chopped

- 1 tablespoon extra-virgin olive oil

- juice of 1 / 4 lemon

- 1 / 4 cup (10g) parsley, chopped

Instructions:

1. Place the salad leaves on a plate or in a large bowl.

2. Mix all the remaining ingredients together and serve on top of the leaves.

Variations:

- Replace the smoked salmon with 1 1 / 3 cup (100g) canned green lentils or cooked Le Puy lentils for a lentil Sirt super salad.

- Replace the smoked salmon with a sliced fried chicken breast for a chicken Sirt super salad.

- According to preference, simply substitute the smoked salmon with canned tuna (in water or oil) for a tuna Sirt super salad.

11.   Char-grilled beef with a red wine jus, onion rings, garlic kale, and herb-roasted potatoes

(Serving: 1, Cooking time: 30 Minutes, Difficulty: Normal)

Ingredients:

- 1 / 2 cup (100g) potatoes, peeled and cut into 3 / 4 -inch (2cm) diced pieces

- 1 tablespoon extra-virgin olive oil

- 2 tablespoons (5g) parsley, finely chopped

- 1 / 3 cup (50g) red onion, sliced into rings

- 2 ounces (50g) kale, sliced

- 2 garlic cloves, finely chopped

- 1 x 4- to 5-ounce (120 to 150g) beef tenderloin (about 1 1 / 2 inch or 3.5cm thick) or sirloin steak (3 / 4 inch or 2cm thick)

- 3 tablespoons (40ml) red wine

- 5 / 8 cup (150ml) beef stock

- 1 teaspoon tomato purée

- 1 teaspoon corn flour, dissolved in

- 1 tablespoon water

Instructions:

1. Heat the oven to 2200C (4250F). Place the potatoes in a boiling water saucepan, bring to a boil again and simmer for 4 to 5 minutes, then drain. Put 1-teaspoon of oil in the roasting pan and roast for 35 to 45 minutes in the hot oven. Switch the potatoes and make sure they cook evenly after 10 minutes.

2. Remove from the oven until baked, sprinkle with chopped parsley, and blend properly. Over medium heat, fry the onion in 1 teaspoon of oil for 5 to 7 minutes, until soft and nicely caramelized. Just stay wet. For 2 to 3 minutes, steam the kale, then rinse. Gently fry the garlic in 1/2 teaspoon of oil, until soft but not browned, for 1 minute. Attach the kale and fry for an extra 1 to 2 minutes, until tender. Just stay wet.

3. Over high pressure, heat an ovenproof frying pan before you smoke. Coat the meat in 1/2 teaspoon of the oil and fry it over medium-high heat in the hot pan as you want the meat done (see our cooking time guide). It would be easier to sear it and then move the pan to an oven set at 4250F (2200C) if you prefer the meat medium and finish the cooking that way for the specified times.

4. Set aside to rest and remove the meat from the pan. To put in some meat residue, add the wine to the hot pan. Simmer to decrease the wine by half until the wine is syrupy and tastes concentrated. In the steak pan, add the stock and tomato purée and bring to a boil, then add the paste of corn-flour to thicken

the sauce, adding it a little at a time until you get the consistency you like.

5. Stir in any of the juices from the rested steak, and serve with the roasted potatoes, kale, onion rings, and red wine sauce.

12.   Kidney bean mole with baked potato

(Serving: 1, Cooking time: 25 Minutes, Difficulty: Normal)

Ingredients:

- 1 / 4 cup (40g) red onion, finely chopped
- 1 teaspoon finely chopped fresh ginger
- 2 garlic cloves, finely chopped
- 1 Thai chili, finely chopped
- 1 teaspoon extra-virgin olive oil
- 1 teaspoon ground turmeric
- 1 teaspoon ground cumin pinch of ground clove pinch of ground cinnamon
- 1 medium baking potato
- 7 / 8 cup (190g) canned chopped tomatoes
- 1 teaspoon brown sugar
- 1 / 3 cup (50g) red bell pepper, cored, seeds removed, and roughly chopped
- 5 / 8 cup (150ml) vegetable stock
- 1 tablespoon cocoa powder
- 1 teaspoon sesame seeds

- 2 teaspoons peanut butter (smooth if available, but chunky is fine)

- 7 / 8 cup (150) canned kidney beans

- 2 tablespoons (5g) parsley, chopped

Instructions:

1. Heat the oven to 200oC (400°F). In a medium saucepan over medium heat, fry the onion, ginger, garlic, and chili in the oil for about 10 minutes until tender. Attach the seasoning, then simmer for 1 to 2 more minutes.

2. Place the potato in the hot oven on a baking tray and bake for 45 to 60 minutes, until the middle is soft (or longer, depending on how crispy the outside maybe).

3. Meanwhile, add to the saucepan the tomatoes, cinnamon, red pepper, stock, cocoa powder, sesame seeds, peanut butter, and kidney beans and gently simmer for 45 to 60 minutes. To end, sprinkle with the parsley.

5. Break the potato in half and serve on top with the mole.

13.   Sirtfood Omelet

(Serving: 1, Cooking time: 20 Minutes, Difficulty: Normal)

Ingredients:

- 2 ounces (50g) sliced streaky bacon (or 2 rashers, smoked or regular, depending on your taste) 3 medium eggs

- 1 1 / 4-ounces (35g) red endive, thinly sliced

- 2 tablespoons (5g) parsley, finely chopped

- 1 teaspoon turmeric

- 1 teaspoon extra-virgin olive oil

Instructions:

1. Heat a frying pan with a nonstick. Break the bacon into thin strips and fry until crispy over high heat.

2. There is enough fat in the bacon to fry it, so you don't need to add any grease. Remove from the pan and put to drain some extra fat on a paper towel. Wipe in a clean bath. Whisk together the eggs and blend with the turmeric, parsley, and endives.

3. Chop the fried bacon into small cubes and stir in the eggs. In the frying pan, heat the oil; the pan should be hot but not burning. Apply the egg mixture and move it around the pan using a spatula to start cooking the egg.

4. Keep the cooked egg bits going and rotate around the pan with the raw egg until the omelet level is even. Reduce the heat and let it firm up the omelet.

5. Ease along the spatula's sides and fold the omelet in half or roll up and serve.

14. Baked chicken breast with walnut and parsley pesto and red onion salad

(Serving: 1, Cooking time: 35 Minutes, Difficulty: Normal)

Ingredients:

- 3 / 8 cup (15g) parsley 1 / 8 cup (15g) walnuts

- 4 teaspoons (15g) Parmesan cheese, grated

- 1 tablespoon extra-virgin olive oil

- juice of 1 / 2 lemon

- 3 tablespoons (50ml) water

- 5 1 / 2 ounces (150g) skinless chicken breast

- 1 / 8 cup (20g) red onions, finely sliced

- 1 teaspoon red wine vinegar

- 1 1 / 4-ounces (35g) arugula

- 2 / 3 cup (100g) cherry tomatoes, halved

- 1 teaspoon balsamic vinegar

Instructions:

1. Place the parsley, walnuts, parmesan, olive oil, half of the lemon juice and a little water in a food processor or blender to make the pesto and mix until the paste is smooth. Gradually, add more water until you have your desired consistency.

2. Marinate 1-tablespoon of the pesto with the chicken breast and the remaining lemon juice in the fridge for 30 minutes, if possible, longer. Preheat your oven to 2000C (4000F). Over medium-high prepare, heat an ovenproof frying pan.

3. Fry the chicken on either side for 1 minute in its marinade, then move the pan to the oven and roast for 8 minutes or until fully fried. For 5 to 10 minutes, marinate the onions in the red wine vinegar. Drain the fluid.

3. Remove it from the oven when the chicken is baked, spoon another pesto tablespoon over it and let the heat from the chicken melt the pesto.

4. Cover with foil and leave to rest before serving for 5 minutes. Combine the cabbage, tomatoes, and arugula and drizzle the balsamic vinegar with it.

5. Serve with the chicken and spoon the remaining pesto over it.

15.   **Waldorf salad**

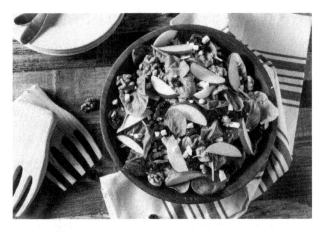

(Serving: 1, Cooking time: 20 Minutes, Difficulty: Normal)

Ingredients:

- 1 cup (100g) celery including leaves, roughly chopped

- 1 / 2 cup (50g) apple, roughly chopped

- 3 / 8 cup (50g) walnuts, roughly chopped

- 1 tablespoon (10g) red onion, roughly chopped

- 2 tablespoons (5g) parsley, chopped

- 1 tablespoon capers

- 1 tablespoon extra-virgin olive oil

- 1 teaspoon balsamic vinegar

- juice of 1 / 4 lemon 1 / 4 teaspoon Dijon mustard

- 2 ounces (50g) arugula about 1

- 1 / 2 ounces (35g) endive leaves

Instructions:

1. Mix the celery and its leaves, apple, walnuts, and onion with the parsley and capers. In a bowl, whisk the oil, vinegar, lemon juice, and mustard to make the dressing.

2. Serve the celery mixture on top of the arugula and endive and drizzle with the dressing.

16. Roasted eggplant wedges with walnut and parsley pesto and tomato salad

(Serving: 1, Cooking time: 25 Minutes, Difficulty: Normal)

Ingredients:

- 1 / 2 cup (20g) parsley

- 3 / 4 ounces (20g) walnuts

- 1 / 8 cup (20g)

- Parmesan cheese (or use a vegetarian or vegan alternative), grated

- 1 tablespoon extra-virgin olive oil

- juice of 1 / 4 lemon

- 3 tablespoons (50ml) water

- 1 small eggplant (around 5 1 / 2 ounces or 150g), quartered

- 1 / 8 cup (20g) red onions, sliced

- 1 teaspoon (5ml) red wine vinegar

- 1 1 / 4-ounces (35g) arugula

- 2 / 3 cup (100g) cherry tomatoes

- 1 teaspoon (5ml) balsamic vinegar

Instructions:

1. Heat the oven to around 200oC (400oF). Place the parsley, walnuts, parmesan, olive oil, and half the lemon juice in a food processor mixer to make the pesto and blend until the paste is smooth.

2. Add the water steadily until you have the right consistency. To adhere to the eggplant, it should be thick enough. Brush some of the pesto with the eggplant, reserving the remainder to serve. Place on a baking sheet and cook for 25 to 30 minutes, until the eggplant becomes brown, delicate, and damp.

3. Meanwhile, cover and set aside the red onion with the red wine vinegar, softening and sweetening the onion.

4. Before serving, drain the vinegar. Combine the tomatoes, arugula, and drained onion and drizzle over the salad with the balsamic vinegar.

5. Serve with the hot eggplant and spoon over it with the remaining pesto.

17. Sirtfood Smoothie

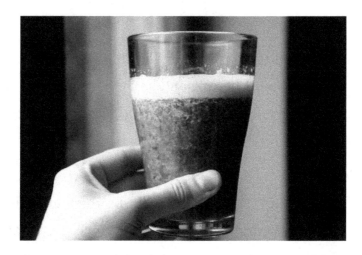

(Serving: 1, Cooking time: 35 Minutes, Difficulty: Normal)

Ingredients:

- 3 / 8 cup (100g) plain Greek yogurt (or vegan alternative, such as soy or coconut yogurt)

- 6 walnut halves

- 8 to 10 medium strawberries, hulled handful of kale, stalks removed

- 3 / 4 ounce (20g) dark chocolate (85 percent cocoa solids)

- 1 Medjool date, pitted

- 1 / 2 teaspoon ground turmeric thin sliver (1 to 2mm) of Thai chili

- 7 / 8 cup (200ml) unsweetened almond milk

Instructions:

1. Blitz all the ingredients in a blender until smooth.

18.   Stuffed whole-wheat pita

(Serving: 1, Cooking time: 25 Minutes, Difficulty: Normal)

Ingredients:

For a meat option:

- 3 ounces (80g) cooked turkey slices, chopped

- 3 / 4-ounce (20g) cheddar cheese, diced

- 1 / 4 cup (35g) cucumber, diced

- 1 / 4 cup (35g) red onion, chopped

- 1-ounce (25g) arugula, chopped

- 1 1 / 2 to 2 tablespoons (10 to 15g) walnuts, roughly chopped

For the dressing:

- 1 tablespoon extra-virgin olive oil

- 1 tablespoon balsamic vinegar dash of lemon juice

For a vegan option:

- 2 to 3 tablespoons hummus

- 1 / 4 cup (35g) cucumber, diced

- 1 / 4 cup (35g) red onion, chopped

- 1-ounce (25g) arugula, chopped

- 1 1 / 2 to 2 tablespoons (10 to 15g) walnuts, roughly chopped

For the vegan dressing:

- 1 tablespoon extra-virgin olive oil dash of lemon juice.

19.   Butternut squash and date tagine with buckwheat

(Serving: 1, Cooking time: 20 Minutes, Difficulty: Normal)

Ingredients:

- 3 teaspoons extra-virgin olive oil

- 1 red onion, finely chopped

- 1 tablespoon finely chopped fresh ginger

- 4 garlic cloves, finely chopped

- 2 Thai chilies, finely chopped

- 1 tablespoon ground cumin

- 1 cinnamon stick

- 2 tablespoons ground turmeric

- 2 x 14-ounce cans (400g each) of chopped tomatoes

- 1 1 / 4 cup (300ml) vegetable stock

- 2 / 3 cup (100g) Medjool dates, pitted and chopped

- 1 x 14-ounce can (400g) of chickpeas, drained and rinsed

- 2 1 / 2 cups (500g) butternut squash, peeled and cut into bite-size pieces

- 1 1 / 4 cup (200g) buckwheat

- 2 tablespoons (5g) fresh coriander, chopped

- 1 / 4 cup (10g) fresh parsley, chopped

Instructions:

1. Heat the oven to 200oC (400oF). For 2 to 3 minutes, fry the onion, ginger, garlic, and chili in two teaspoons of oil. Add the cumin, cinnamon, 1-tablespoon of turmeric, and simmer for 1 to 2 more minutes.

2. For 45 to 60 minutes, add the tomatoes, stock, dates, and chickpeas and simmer gently. To achieve a thick, moist consistency and make sure the pan does not run dry, you can apply a little water from time to time.

3. In a roasting pan, put the squash, toss with the rest of the oil and roast for 30 minutes until it is tender and crispy around the edges. Cook the buckwheat according to the product directions with turmeric's remaining tablespoon towards the end of the tagine's cooking period.

4. Add the roasted squash along with the cilantro and parsley to the tagine and serve with the buckwheat.

20.   Butter bean and miso dip with celery sticks and oatcakes

(Serving: 1, Cooking time: 20 Minutes, Difficulty: Normal)

Ingredients:

- 2 x 14-ounce cans (400g each) of butter beans, drained and rinsed

- 3 tablespoons extra-virgin olive oil

- 2 tablespoons brown miso paste juice and grated zest of 1 / 2 unwaxed lemon

- 4 medium scallions, trimmed and finely chopped

- 1 garlic clove, crushed

- 1 / 4 Thai chili, finely chopped celery sticks, to serve oatcakes, to serve

Instructions:

1. Simply mash the first seven ingredients together with a potato masher until you have a coarse mixture.

2. Serve as a dip with celery sticks and oatcakes.

CHAPTER 5:

Snacks & Desserts Recipes

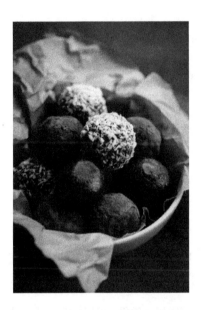

It is imminent that you will feel a pang of hunger at specific points in the day and have the urge to grab a meal. The snack foods and desserts listed as Sirtfood bites will help you relapse to eating unhealthy foods, as they are comfortable, temporarily hold you full and are deliciously enjoyable if you are the type of person who used to eat a lot of junk foods beforehand.

21.   Fried chili tofu

(Serving: 1, Cooking time: 20 minutes, Difficulty: Easy)

Ingredients:

- 150 g firm tofu, cut into cubes
- 1 clove of garlic, peeled and crushed juice of
- ½ lemon
- ½ teaspoon chili flakes
- ½ teaspoon paprika
- ½ teaspoon ground turmeric
- Salt and freshly ground black pepper
- 1 teaspoon oil

Instructions:

1. Spread the tofu on a plate with kitchen paper. Cover with kitchen paper and set aside to dry. Put the garlic, lemon juice, spices, and a generous spice mixture of salt and pepper in a wide bowl.

2. Mix everything together before adding the tofu and mix gently so that the tofu is completely covered.

3. Let stand for 5 to 15 minutes. Heat the oil in a pan over medium-high heat and wait until the pan is hot before removing the tofu from the marinade and adding it to the pan. Fry for 3–4 minutes, stirring every minute, until the tofu is golden brown all over. Turn off the heat, add the remaining marinade to the pan and serve.

22.   Olive tapenade

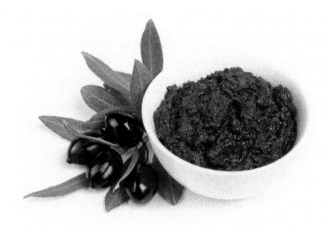

(Serving: 4, Cooking time: 20 minutes, Difficulty: Easy)

Ingredients:

- 1 clove of garlic, peeled and crushed peel

- Juice of ½ lemon

- 1 tbsp capers

- Drain 3 anchovy fillets, chop them up

- Drain 200 g pitted green or black olives and roughly chop

- 2 tbsp extra virgin olive oil

Instructions:

1. Put the garlic, lemon peel and juice, capers and anchovies in a food processor and stir until smooth.

2. Add the olives and mix again. Do not overmix as some pieces of olive will ensure a good consistency. Scoop out the paste and stir in the olive oil. The tapenade stays in the refrigerator for a few days.

23.   Crispy fried olives

(Serving: 2, Cooking time: 20 minutes, Difficulty: Easy)

Ingredients:

- 200 g green pitted olives

- 1 egg, beaten

- 50 g panko breadcrumbs

- ½ teaspoon ground turmeric

- ½ teaspoon paprika

- 1 tbsp olive oil

Instructions:

1. Dry the olives on paper towels. Place the beaten eggs in a shallow bowl and mix the breadcrumbs, turmeric, and peppers in another.

2. Dip and coat the olives in the beaten egg first, then roll in the breadcrumbs.

3. Heat the oil in a wide pan over medium heat. When hot, add the coated olives and saute until golden brown all over.

4. Remove with a slotted spoon and drain on kitchen paper before serving.

24.   Turmeric apple chips

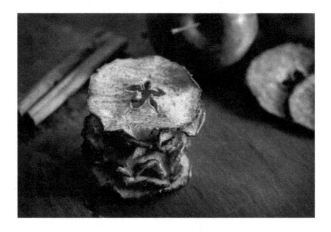

(Serving: 2-3, Cooking time: 1 Hour, Difficulty: Normal)

Ingredients:

- Juice of ½ lemon   ¼ teaspoon ground turmeric

- ½ teaspoon ground cinnamon

- ½ teaspoon ground ginger

- 1 large apple

Instructions:

1. Preheat the oven (100 ° C fan/gas ½) to 120 ° C. Using parchment paper or silicone sheets to cover two baking sheets. In a shallow bowl, add the lemon juice and mix in the spices.

2. Break the top of the apple off. Cut tiny apple circles over the top with the aid of a peeler. The seeds in the centre are all coming out.

3. Drop it into the lemon juice as each skinny slice has peeled off, then lightly mix more lemon juice over it to prevent browning. Discard the apple foundation. Arrange the apple rings over the baking sheets in one layer. Bake for 1 hour and 15 minutes, then change around for 45 minutes.

5. Take out of the oven and let cool on the baking sheet before storing in an airtight container.

25.   Chocolate treat

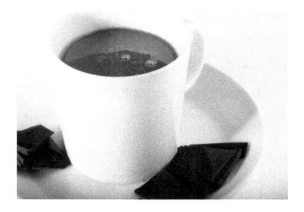

(Serving: 2, Cooking time: 10 minutes, Difficulty: Easy)

Ingredients:

- 2 heaped teaspoons (20 g) high quality cocoa powder
- 2 tsp (10 g) granulated sugar
- Some boiling water
- 60 ml of milk

Instructions:

1. Put the cocoa and sugar in a small jug. Add a little water from the kettle, just enough to make a smooth paste.

2. Pour in the milk one at a time, stirring thoroughly. Pour into two shot glasses and enjoy your chocolate hit straight away.

26.   Frozen chocolate grapes

(Serving: 4, Cooking time: 15 minutes, Difficulty: Easy)

Ingredients:

- 50 g good quality dark chocolate (70%)
- 150 g red seedless grapes

Instructions:

1. Line a silicone layer or baking paper with a baking sheet. Break the chocolate into little bits and put it in a small, heat-resistant bowl. Heat a small pan of water, gently boil and put the chocolate bowl on it. Make sure the water should not hit the bowl.

2. Heat and mix the chocolate so that it melts slowly, and if there are lumps left, remove it from the heat. Keep the chocolate stirring until it is molten (this will stop white spots or blooms on the chocolate).

3. One by one, dip the grapes in the chocolate to be half-coated and put them on the baking sheet immediately. For all the grapes, continue. Before throwing it in the fridge, let the chocolate harden at room temperature. The grapes may be stored in an adequate freezer jar after freezing.

4. Serve in servings of 10 to 12 grapes at a time, or just reach in and take a few if needed.

27.　　Chocolate Matcha Energy balls

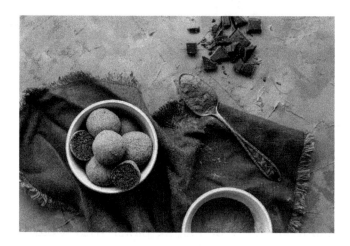

(Serving: 10, Cooking time: 20 minutes, Difficulty: Easy)

Ingredients:

- 100 g soft dates

- 100 g blanched almonds

- 50 g high quality cocoa powder

- 1 tbsp matcha green tea powder + more to refine

- 2 tbsp almond milk

Instructions:

1. Place the dates and almonds in a food processor and process them until they come together into a sticky ball. With a fork, crack open the ball and add chocolate, matcha and almond milk.

2. Mix before a big sticky ball emerges. Please take out the mixture with big, heaping teaspoons and roll them into small compact balls.

3. Repeat until there are 10 or 12 balls for you. Dust over a bit more powdered matcha. For up to 2 weeks, these balls remain refrigerated.

28.   Apples and Plum Cake

(Servings: 4 Cook time: 50 minutes, Difficulty: Normal)

Ingredients:

- 7 oz. almond flour 1 egg, whisked

- 5 tablespoons stevia

- 3 oz. warm almond milk

- 2 lbs. plums, pitted and cut into quarters

- 2 apples, cored and chopped

- Zest of 1 lemon, grated

- 1 tsp. baking powder

Instructions:

1. In a bowl, mix the almond milk with the egg, stevia, and the rest of the ingredients except the cooking spray and whisk well.

2. Grease a cake pan with the oil, pour the cake mix inside, introduce in the oven and bake at 350°F for 40 minutes. 3. Cool down, slice and serve.

29.   Baked pomegranate Cheesecake

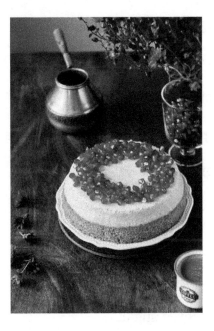

(Serving: 12, Cooking time: 1-2 Hours, Difficulty: Normal)

Ingredients:

For the crust:

- 200 g pistachios

- 50 g powdered sugar

- ½ teaspoon ground cardamom

- 50 g melted butter

For the filling:

- 500 g cream cheese

- 200 g powdered sugar

- 30 g milk powder

- 30 grams of flour

- 300 ml sour cream

- 2 eggs, separated   2 tsp vanilla bean paste

- 3 sheets of gelatine

- 125 ml of water

For covering:

- 250 ml pomegranate juice

- 1 tbsp powdered sugar

- 4 sheets of gelatine

- 150 g pomegranate seeds

Instructions:

1. Preheat the oven to 170 ° C (150 ° C fan / gas 3).

2. Line a large, loose-bottomed, straight-sided cake pan on the bottom with a piece of baking paper. Finely chop the pistachios, sugar and cardamom with a food processor. Pour in the melted butter and combine them into a paste. Press into the bottom of the prepared pan and bake for 8 minutes. Set aside to cool. In a blender or by hand, stir the cream cheese and powdered sugar until creamy. Add milk powder and flour and mix well.

3. Add sour cream, egg yolks and vanilla. Dissolve the gelatin in the water according to the instructions in the package and then add to the cheesecake filling while stirring well. In a clean bowl, beat the egg whites until light and fluffy. Carefully fold into the filling mixture. Rub the sides of the cooled cake pan with some butter then add the cheesecake filling.

4. Place the can on a large sheet of foil and crumple the foil around the sides of the can. Take a roasting tray and fill it with 5 cm of hot water. Place the cheesecake in the tray and bake it in the oven for about 1 hour (still at 170 ° C / 150 ° C fan / gas 3). Turn off the oven and let it cool in the oven for an additional hour (this should prevent it from cracking) before allowing it to cool completely at room temperature. Heat the pomegranate juice until it is warm but not bubbly. Stir in the sugar until it has dissolved.

5. Assemble the gelatine according to the instructions in the package and add to the pomegranate juice. Let cool down to room temperature. Pour about a third of the pomegranate over the cheesecake and refrigerate for 10 minutes. Repeat with the next third of the juice and refrigerate for another 10 minutes. Finally, pour the last third of the juice over it, smooth it out with the back of a spoon and spread the pomegranate seeds over it. Cover and refrigerate again for 4 hours.

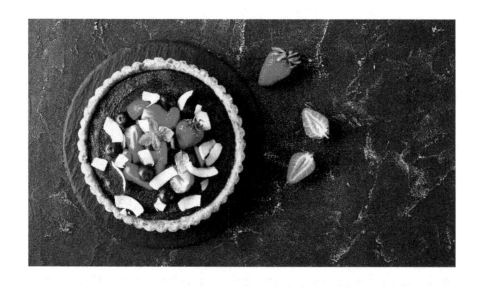

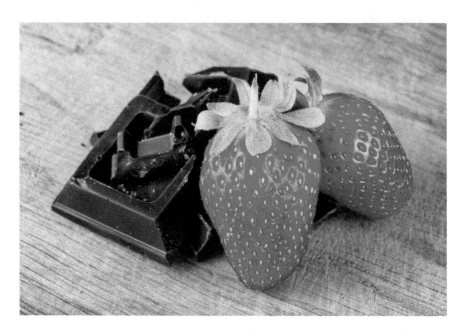

CHAPTER 6:

Beverages & Drinks

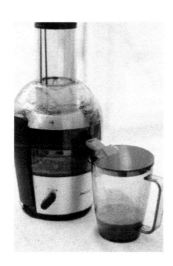

Incredible sirtfood drinks recipes that can hopefully be made for a perfect balanced drink.

30.　Classic Sirt juice

(Serving: 1 Cooking time: 15 Minutes, Difficulty: Easy)

Ingredients:

- 2 handfuls (75 g) kale Handful (30g) arugula

- 5 g parsley 150 g green celery (2-3 stalks)

- ½ green apple ½ lemon - juiced

- ½ teaspoon matcha powder (green tea)

Instructions:

1. Juice ingredients, should have made 250ml (1 cup) once enough for 1 juice.

2. Add matcha powder, shake or stir to combine and drink.

31.   Go green smoothie

(Serving: 1 Cooking time: 15 Minutes, Difficulty: Easy)

Ingredients:

- 200 ml orange juice
- ¼ cucumber with skin
- 1 great property of kale
- 1 prize cinnamon
- 1 apple
- 1 piece of ginger
- 1 pear

Instructions:

1. Mix all ingredients smoothly and serve.

32.   Juicy smoothie

(Serving: 1 Cooking time: 15 Minutes, Difficulty: Normal)

Ingredients:

- 150 ml of water or coconut water

- 1 slice of lemon with peel

- 1 banana

- 1 large key spinach

- 1 apple Juice of 1 orange

- ¼ avocado without stone

Instructions:

1. Mix all ingredients smoothly and serve.

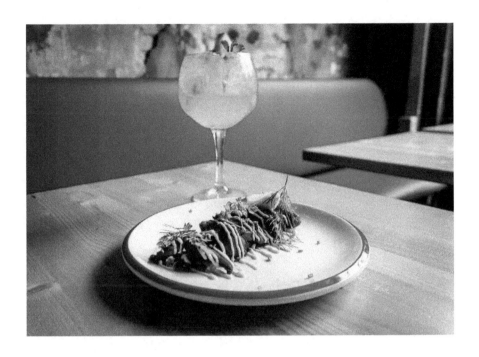

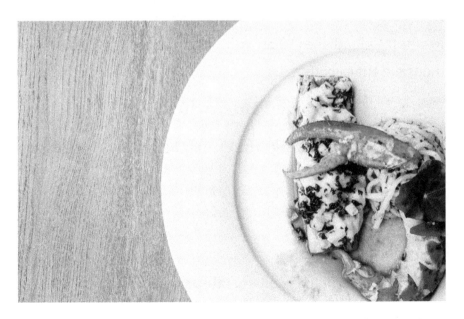

CHAPTER 7:

Side Dish Recipes

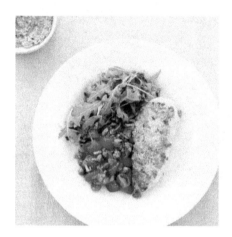

Recipes Side dishes that will make weeknight dinners a thousand times better.

33.   Egg Fried Buckwheat

(Serving: 6, Cooking time: 10 Minutes, Difficulty: Easy)

Ingredients:

- Eggs, beaten – 2

- Extra virgin olive oil – 2 tablespoons, divided

- Onion, diced – 1

- Peas, frozen - .5 cup

- Carrots, finely diced – 2

- Garlic, minced – 2 cloves

- Ginger, grated – 1 teaspoon

- Green onions, thinly sliced – 2

- Tamari sauce – 2 tablespoons

- Sriracha sauce – 2 teaspoons

- Cooked buckwheat groats, cold – 3 cups

Instructions:

1. Add half of the olive oil to a large skillet or wok set to medium heat and add in the egg, stirring constantly until it is fully cooked. Remove the egg and transfer it to another dish.

2. Add the remaining olive oil to your wok along with the peas, carrots, and onion. Cook until the carrots and onions are softened, about four minutes. Add in the grated ginger and minced garlic, cooking for an additional minute until fragrant.

3. Add the sriracha sauce, tamari sauce, and cooked buckwheat groats to the wok. Continue to cook the buckwheat groats and stir the mixture until the buckwheat is warmed all the way through and the flavours have melded, about two minutes.

4. Add the cooked eggs and green onions to the wok, giving it a good toss to combine and serve warm.

34. Aromatic Ginger Turmeric Buckwheat

(Serving: 4, Cooking time: 25 Minutes, Difficulty: Normal)

kilocalories Per Individual Serving: 285 The Number of Servings: 4 Time to Prepare/Cook: 25 minutes

Ingredients:

- Buckwheat groats, rinsed and drained – 1 cup

- Water – 1.75 cup Extra virgin olive oil – 1 tablespoon

- Ginger, grated – 1 tablespoon

- Garlic, minced – 3 cloves

- Turmeric root, grated – 1 teaspoon

- Lemon juice – 1 tablespoon

- Sea salt – 1 teaspoon

- Cranberries, dried - .5 cup

- Parsley, chopped - .33 cup

- Pine nuts, toasted - .25 cup (optional)

Instructions:

1. Into a medium saucepan add the buckwheat groats, water, olive oil, ginger, garlic, turmeric, lemon juice, and sea salt. Bring the water in the pot to a boil and then cover the mixture

with a lid. Allow it to simmer over medium-low until all of the liquid is absorbed, about twenty minutes.

2. About fifteen minutes into the cooking time of the buckwheat sir the dried cranberries into the buckwheat, allowing them to plump up the last few minutes of the cooking time.

3. Top the buckwheat with the pine nuts and parsley before serving.

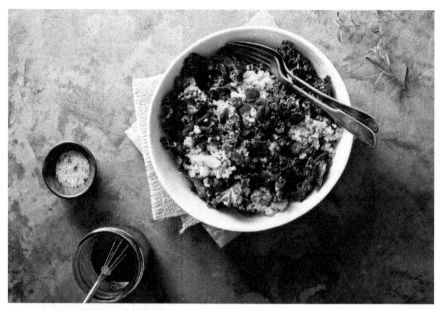

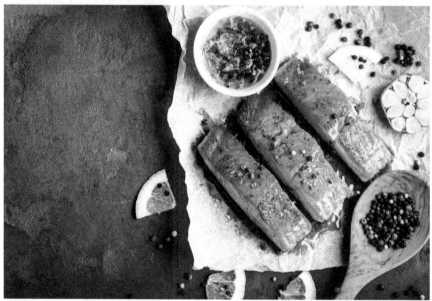

CHAPTER 8:

Salad and Dressing Recipes

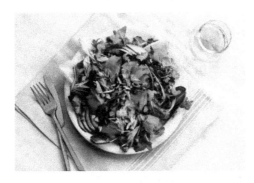

We'll cover some interesting SIRT salad recipes in this chapter. SIRT Salad Recipes can be an enjoyable way to eat vegetables and fruits daily.

35. Buckwheat and Broccoli Salad in Tangy Miso Dressing

(Serving: 5, Cooking time: 40 Minutes, Difficulty: Normal)

Ingredients:

- 1 cup buckwheat groats

- 1½ cups water

- 2 tablespoons red miso

- 1 tablespoon canola oil 1 tablespoon rice vinegar

- 1 tablespoon dark sesame oil

- 1 tablespoon grated ginger

- 1 clove garlic, minced or crushed

- ¼ teaspoon red pepper flakes

- 1 tablespoon honey

- 2 cups broccoli florets, blanched

- ½ cup julienned carrot

- 2 scallions, minced

- ½ cup cashews, toasted

Instructions:

1. In a small, heavy saucepan, heat the buckwheat groats over medium high temperature. Swirl the groats in the pan, toasting them until they are crackling, hot to the touch, and fragrant, about 5 minutes. In a wiremesh strainer, wash the hot buckwheat q uickly and drain thoroughly.

2. Put the 1½ cups water in the pan and bring to a boil. Add the buckwheat, return to a boil, cover tightly, and reduce the heat to the lowest setting. Cook for about 20 minutes, until all the liquid is absorbed. Take the pan off the heat and let stand for 5 minutes, then transfer the cooked grain to a bowl, cover, and let cool to room temperature.

3. In a large measuring cup, whisk the miso, canola oil, and vinegar until smooth. Whisk in the sesame oil, ginger, garlic, pepper flakes, and honey. Pour the dressing over the cooled buckwheat and toss to coat.

4. To serve, spread the buckwheat on a platter, and top with the broccoli, carrot, and scallions. Sprinkle the cashews over the salad and serve. Alternatively, mix the veggies into the grain and chill.

36.   Massaged Kale Salad

(Serving: 4, Cooking time: 20 Minutes, Difficulty: Normal)

Ingredients:

- 1 bunch kale (black kale is especially good), stalks removed and discarded, leaves thinly sliced

- 1 lemon, juiced

- 1/4 cup extra-virgin olive oil, plus extra for drizzling Kosher salt

- 2 teaspoons honey

- Freshly ground black pepper

- 1 mango, diced small (about 1 cup)

- Small handful toasted pepitas (pumpkin seeds), about 2 rounded tablespoons

Instructions:

1. In large serving bowl, add the kale, half of lemon juice, a drizzle of oil and a little kosher salt. Massage until the kale starts to soften and wilt, 2 to 3 minutes. Set aside while you make the dressing. In a small bowl, whisk remaining lemon juice with the honey and lots of freshly ground black pepper. Stream in the 1/4 cup of oil while whisking until a dressing

forms, and you like how it tastes. Pour the dressing over the kale, and add the mango and pepitas. Toss and serve.

Nutrition: Calories: 198 Total Fat: 13g Saturated Fat: 5g Cholesterol: 0mg Sodium: 230mg Carbohydrates: 3g

37. Baked Salmon Salad with Creamy Mint Dressing

(Serving: 1, Cooking time: 30 Minutes, Difficulty: Normal)

Ingredients:

- 1 salmon fillet (130g)

- 40g mixed salad leaves

- 40g young spinach leaves

- 2 radishes, trimmed and thinly sliced

- 5cm piece (50g) cucumber, cut into chunks

- 2 spring onions, trimmed and sliced

- 1 small handful (10g) parsley, roughly chopped

For the dressing:

- 1 tsp low-fat mayonnaise

- 1 tbsp natural yogurt

- 1 tbsp rice vinegar

- 2 leaves mint, finely chopped

- Salt and freshly ground black pepper

Instructions:

1. Preheat the oven to 200°C (180°C fan/Gas 6).

2. Place the salmon fillet on a baking tray and bake for 16–18 minutes until just cooked through. Remove from the oven and set aside. The salmon is equally nice hot or cold in the salad. If your salmon has skin, simply cook skin side down and remove the salmon from the skin using a fish slice after cooking. It should slide off easily when cooked.

3. In a small bowl, mix together the mayonnaise, yogurt, rice wine vinegar, mint leaves and salt and pepper together and leave to stand for at least 5 minutes to allow the flavors to develop.

4. Arrange the salad leaves and spinach on a serving plate and top with the radishes, cucumber, spring onions and parsley. Flake the cooked salmon onto the salad and drizzle the dressing over.

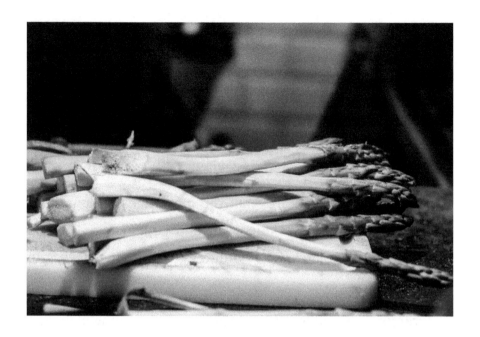

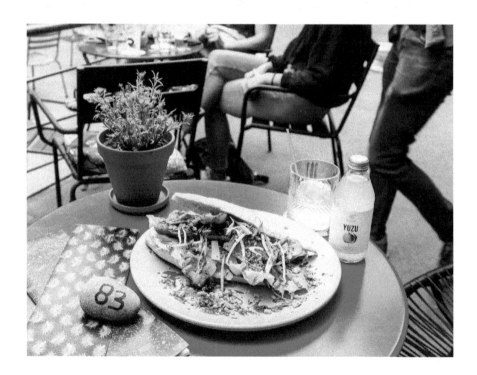

CHAPTER 9:

Fast Meal Recipes

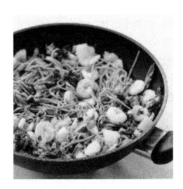

SIRT Meal Recipes will Take Your Breath away. Try Short Meal and essential recipes of Sirtfood full of flavour and goodness.

38.   Fresh Saag Paneer

(Serving: 2, Cooking time: 10 Minutes, Difficulty: Normal)

Ingredients:

- 2 teaspoons of rapeseed oil

- 200 g paneer, cut into cubes

- Salt and freshly ground black pepper

- 1 red onion, chopped

- 1 small thumb (3 cm) fresh ginger, peeled and cut into matches 1 clove of garlic, peeled and thinly sliced

- 1 green chili, pitted

- 100 g cherry tomatoes sliced, halved

- ½ teaspoon ground coriander

- ½ teaspoon ground cumin

- ¼ teaspoon ground turmeric

- ½ teaspoon mild chili powder

- ½ teaspoon salt

- 100 g fresh spinach leaves

- small handful (10 g) parsley, chopped

- Small handful (10 g) coriander, chopped

Instructions:

1. Heat the oil in a pan with a wide lid over high heat. Season the paneer generously with salt and pepper and add to the pan. Fry for a few minutes until golden brown, stirring frequently. Remove from pan with a slotted spoon and set aside.

2. Reduce the heat and add the onion. Fry for 5 minutes before adding the ginger, garlic and chili. Let simmer for a few minutes before adding the cherry tomatoes. Put the lid on the pan and cook for another 5 minutes.

3. Add the spices and salt and stir. Place the paneer back in the pan and stir until coated. Put the spinach in the pan with the parsley and coriander and put the lid on.

4. Let the spinach wilt for 1–2 minutes, then add it to the bowl. Serve immediately.

39. Teriyaki salmon with Chinese vegetables

(Serving: 2, Cooking time: 15 Minutes, Difficulty: Normal)

Ingredients:

- 1 thumb (5 cm) fresh ginger, peeled and grated
- 1 tbsp soy sauce
- 1 teaspoon fish sauce
- 1 teaspoon honey
- 1 teaspoon sesame oil
- 2 salmon fillets, skinless, quartered
- 1 shallot, peeled and thinly sliced
- ½ carrot, peeled and cut into sticks
- 1 onion of fennel, thinly sliced
- 1 onion pak choi, cut
- 100g kale leaves, stems removed and torn

Instructions:

1. In a large bowl, stir together the ginger, soy, fish sauce, honey and sesame oil.

2. Place the salmon pieces in the bowl, turn them and cover each piece with the sauce.

3. Let it rest while you prepare the rest of the meal. In a large pan with a lid, add about 5 mm - 1 cm of water and bring to the boil.

4. Add the shallot, carrot and fennel. Put the lid on the pan and cook for 4 minutes.

5. Add the pak choi and kale, stir gently and add a little more water when the pan looks dry.

6. Place the salmon pieces on top of the vegetables and pour in the remaining marinade. Put the lid back on the pan and steam for 8 minutes, until the salmon is cooked through.

40.   Kale tomatoes Pasta

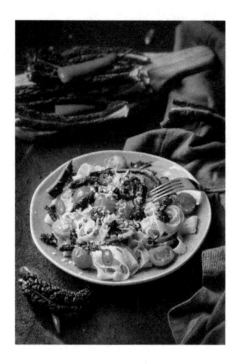

(Serving: 2, Cooking time: 20 Minutes, Difficulty: Normal)

Ingredients:

- 200 g linguine

- 200 g cherry tomatoes, halved lemon zest

- Juice of ½ lemon

- 50 ml of extra-virgin olive oil

- 1 heaped teaspoon sea salt

- 500 ml of boiling water

- 200 g kale leaves, stems removed and roughly torn

- Large handful (20 g) parsley, finely chopped

- 20 g parmesan, finely grated

- Freshly ground black pepper

Instructions:

1. Use a large, shallow pan with a lid wide enough to hold the linguine flat. Add the pasta, tomatoes, lemon zest, lemon juice, olive oil and salt to the pan.

2. Pour over 500 ml of boiling water, put the lid on and bring it to a boil. Once it boils, remove the lid and stir. Continue to cook and stir every minute for 6 minutes.

3. Add the kale and cook for another 2 minutes or until almost all of the water has evaporated.

4. Combine the parsley, parmesan and black pepper in a small bowl. Divide the pasta between two bowls and sprinkle the parsley and parmesan mixture on top.

CHAPTER 10:

Quick and Easy Recipes

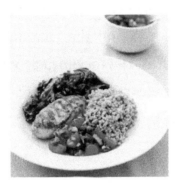

Try Quick and Easy Sirtfood recipes packed with flavour and goodness

41.   Smoked Salmon Omelette

(Serving: 2, Cooking time: 10-20 Minutes, Difficulty: Normal)

Ingredients:

- 2 Medium eggs 100 g Smoked salmon, cut

- 1/2 tsp Capers

- 10 g Rocket, cleaved

- 1 tsp Parsley, cleaved

- 1 tsp Extra-virgin olive oil

Instructions:

1. Break the eggs into a bowl and whisk well. Include the salmon, tricks, rocket and parsley.

2. Warmth the olive oil in a non-stick pan until hot yet not smoking. Include the egg blend and, utilizing a spatula or fish cut, move the blend around the container until it is even. Decrease the warmth and let the omelet cook through. Slide the spatula around the edges and move up or crease the omelet into equal parts to serve.

42. Green Tea Smoothie

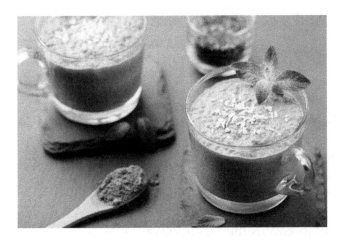

(Serving: 2, Cooking time: 20 Minutes, Difficulty: Normal)

Ingredients:

- 2 ready bananas

- 250 ml milk

- 2 tsp matcha green tea powder

- 1/2 tsp vanilla bean paste (not extricate) or a little scratch of the seeds from a vanilla unit

- 6 ice cubes

- 2 tsp nectar

Instructions:

Mix all the ingredients in a blender and serve in two glasses.

1. Sirt food miso marinated cod with stir-fried greens & sesame

(Serving: 1, Cooking time: 30 Minutes, Difficulty: Normal)

Ingredients:

- 20g miso

- 1 tbsp mirin

- 1 tbsp additional virgin olive oil

- 200g skinless cod filet

- 20g red onion, cut

- 40g celery, cut

- 1 garlic clove, finely hacked

- 1 10,000-foot bean stew, finely hacked

- 1 tsp finely hacked new ginger

- 60g green beans

- 50g kale, generally hacked

- 1 tsp sesame seeds

- 5g parsley, generally hacked

- 1 tbsp tamari

- 30g buckwheat

- 1 tsp ground turmeric

Instructions:

1. Blend the miso, mirin, and 1 teaspoon of the oil. Rub everywhere throughout the cod and leave to marinate for 30 minutes. Warmth the oven to 220°C/gas 7.

2. Heat the cod for 10 minutes.

3. In the meantime, heat a huge pan or wok with the rest of the oil. Include the onion and pan-fried food for a couple of moments, at that point include the celery, garlic, stew, ginger, green beans, and kale. Hurl and fry until the kale is delicate

and cooked through. You may need to add a little water to the dish to help the cooking procedure.

4. Cook the buckwheat as per the bundle guidelines with the turmeric for 3 minutes.

5. Include the sesame seeds, parsley, and tamari to the pan-fried food and present with the greens and fish.

6. Regardless of whether you're attempting to shed pounds or getting progressively careful about energizing your body, it's imperative to comprehend Sirtfoods. Sirtfoods are a group of nourishments wealthy in supplements that help manage your digestion, consume fat, and increment muscle.

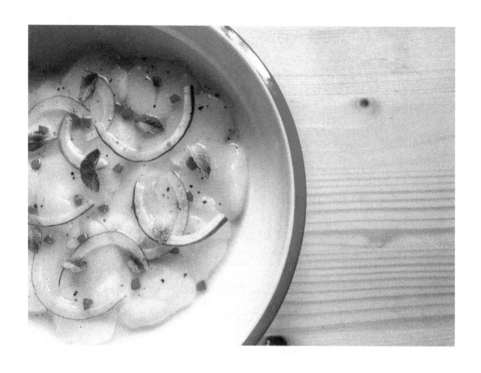

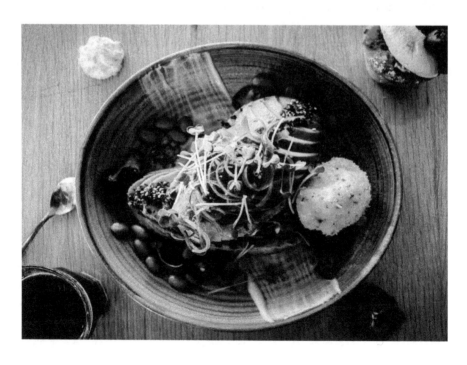

CHAPTER 11:

Light Bite Recipes

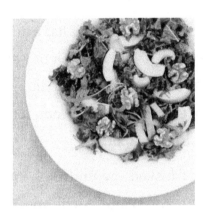

Try Light Recipes Sirtfood recipes packed with flavour and goodness.

2. Kale, Tomato, Spring Onion & Pea Omelette

(Serving: 1, Cooking time: 15 Minutes, Difficulty: Normal)

Ingredients:

- 2 eggs whisked with a splash of milk

- 2 large kale leaves washed, stems removed, shredded

- 1/2 cup frozen peas

- 5 cherry tomatoes washed, halved

- 4 spring onions ends removed, washed, chopped

- 1 TBSP balsamic vinegar

Instructions:

1. As mentioned, prepare all of the ingredients.

2. In a medium-sized frying pan that has a lid, position the kale. Apply the kale to the pan with a splash of water and put the lid firmly. Cook for 2-3 mins over low-medium heat. Remove the lid after 2-3 mins, then continue to cook for a minute or until all the excess water has evaporated.

3. Slowly spill the whisked egg uniformly over the pan's base and rotate the pan to ensure equal coverage. Sprinkle the frozen peas, spring onions and dot the tomatoes over the omelette at an appropriate distance. Replace the lid and cook for around 4-5mins or until the egg is cooked through on low-medium heat.

4. As this would roast the eggs on the underside, don't be tempted to crank up the fire. Serve the omelette when still soft, as soon as the eggs are fried. When needed, season with salt & pepper and add a splash of balsamic vinegar.

CHAPTER 12:

Sauces and Dips Recipes

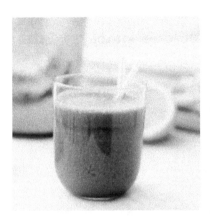

While the largest number of sirtfoods does not include any of these sauces and dips, that's all perfect! The point of these recipes is not to fill up a massive portion of your dinner but merely to bring to your food more flavours and variety. You can find that the sirtfood diet can be varied and tasty with these recipes, while also helping you lose weight and gain fitness.

3. Mango sauce

(Serving: 6, Cooking time: 6 Minutes, Difficulty: Easy)

Ingredients:

- A medium-sized mango

- 2 tablespoons rice vinegar

- Juice of half a lime

- 1 clove of garlic

- 1 tablespoon of red chili

4. Tzatziki

(Serving: 6, Cooking time: 15 Minutes, Difficulty: Easy)

Ingredients:

- 1 clove of garlic

- 150g yogurt

- 10 peppermint leaves

- 1 cucumber

- Juice of one lemon

Instructions:

1. peel and cut the garlic. Roughly grate the cucumber and then squeeze it out so that water is lost.

2. Mix everything together.

CHAPTER 13:

Soup Recipes

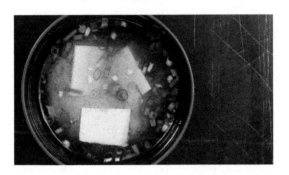

Try SIRT Soup recipes packed with flavour and goodness.

5. Curry broth

(Serving: 4, Cooking time: 25 Minutes, Difficulty: Easy)

Ingredients:

- 1 tbsp olive oil 2 shallots, peeled and finely chopped

- 1 clove of garlic, peeled and finely chopped

- 2 green chilies, pitted and finely chopped

- 1 teaspoon mild chili powder

- 1 teaspoon ground turmeric

- ¼ teaspoon cloves

- ¼ teaspoon ground cinnamon

- 1 teaspoon salt 150 g broccoli, cut into small florets

- 200 g kale leaves, stems removed and roughly chopped

- 400 ml chicken or vegetable stock, fresh

- 1 litre of boiling water

- 250 g tofu, cut into small cubes

- 2 spring onions, cut and chopped

- 20 g coriander, chopped

Instructions:

1. In a large saucepan with a thick bottom, heat the oil over low heat. Add the shallots and saute them for 5 minutes, until they just start to soften.

2. Add the garlic, green chilies, spices, and salt. Stir, then add the broccoli and kale. Fry for 2-3 minutes. Add the stock and water and bring to a boil. Let simmer gently for 15 minutes.

3. Add the tofu, spring onions, and coriander and cook for a few more minutes until it warms up.

CHAPTER 14:

Cake Recipes

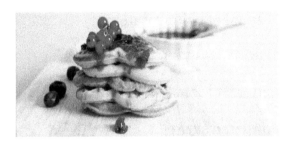

Try Sirtfood Cake recipes packed with flavour and goodness.

6. Chocolate cupcakes with matcha

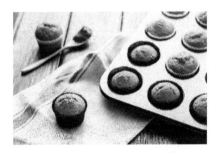

(Serving: 12, Cooking time: 25 Minutes, Difficulty: Normal)

Ingredients:

- 150 g of flour

- 200 g powdered sugar

- 60 g cocoa powder

- ½ teaspoon salt

- ½ tsp fine espresso coffee, if desired

- 120 ml milk ½ teaspoon vanilla extract 50 ml of vegetable oil

- 1 egg 120 ml of boiling water

For the powdered sugar:

- 50 g butter, at room temperature

- 50 g powdered sugar

- 1 tbsp matcha green tea powder

- ½ tsp vanilla bean paste

- 50 g cream cheese

Instructions:

1. Preheat the oven to 180 ° C (160 ° C fan/gas 4).

2. Line a cupcake tin with 12 paper or silicone cake sleeves. Put the flour, sugar, cocoa, salt, and espresso powder in a large bowl and mix well. Add milk, vanilla extract, vegetable oil, and egg to the dry ingredients and mix well with an electric mixer. Gently pour the boiling water slowly and beat on low speed until completely mixed. Use a high-speed beating for another minute to add air to the dough. The batter is much more fluid than a normal cake mix.

3. Spoon the batter evenly into the cake containers. Each cake container should not be more than three-quarters full. Bake in the oven for 15-18 minutes until the mixture bounces back when you tap. Take out of the oven and let cool completely before freezing.

4. For the icing, stir the butter and powdered sugar until they are smooth. Add the matcha powder and vanilla and stir again. Finally, add the cream cheese and stir until smooth.

CHAPTER 15:

Meat and Fish Recipes

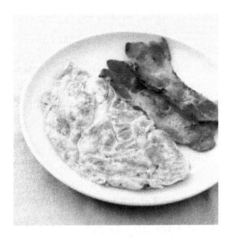

Try Sirtfood Meat and Fish recipes packed with flavour and goodness.

7. Spicy salmon fillet

(Serving: 2, Cooking time: 1 Hour 10 Minutes, Difficulty: Normal)

Ingredients:

- 1 organic lime ¼ tbsp chili powder

- ¼ teaspoon brown sugar

- 1 tbsp olive oil

- 180g salmon fillet

- 1 red pepper

- 50g ripe mango

- ½ red onion

- Coriander, salt, pepper, sugar

Instructions:

1. Squeeze the lime. Rub the peel off one half of the lime.

2. Mix the chili powder, brown sugar, olive oil and 2 tablespoons of lime juice.

3. Put the salmon fillet in the marinade and chill.

4. Quarter and core the peppers and place them on with the skin facing up. Place a baking sheet. Roast under the oven girl until the skin blisters.

5. Put the roasted peppers in a bowl and cover with a plate. Let steam for 10 minutes.

6. Peel the skin off the peppers and cut the pulp into fine diamond pieces.

7. Peel the mango and cut the pulp into equal pieces.

8. peel and finely chop the onion

9. Mix the peppers, mango, onions and coriander with the remaining lime juice and a little olive oil. Season with salt, pepper and a little sugar.

10. Grill the salmon in a grill pan for about 4 minutes on each side.

11.. Arrange the salmon fillet with mango sauce on a plate and enjoy!

8. Lentil soup with porcini mushrooms and duck breast

(Serving: 6, Cooking time: 35 Minutes, Difficulty: Normal)

Ingredients:

- ½ half an onion

- 1 clove of garlic

- 1 tbsp olive oil

- 50g red lentils

- ¼ tbsp tomato paste

- 250ml vegetable stock

- 70g duck breast fillet

- Salt pepper

- 50g porcini mushrooms

- 50 ml soy cream

Instructions:

1. Peel and finely chop the onion and garlic.

2. Steam the onions and garlic in the oil until translucent. Add the lentils and cook with them.

3. Add the tomato market and sauté for 30 seconds. Then add the broth. Bring to a boil and simmer for 15 minutes.

4. Score the duck breast on the skin side, but do not cut into the meat. Sear the breast skin side down in a pan.

5. Turn the duck breast and fry on the meat side for 2-3 minutes—season with salt and pepper. Cover the duck breast with aluminum foil and let it rest for five minutes.

6. clean and chop porcini mushrooms. Fry the mushrooms in oil and season with salt and pepper.

7. puree the soup and add soy cream. Bring to the boil and season with salt and pepper.

8. Cut the duck breast and add it to the soup with the porcini mushrooms.

CONCLUSION

In this book, we have examined, in great detail, the novel and extremely effective sirtfood diet. In the opening chapter, we promised to go over the mechanism of action of the sirtfood diet, the benefits of the diet, the foods that make up the diet, a shopping list for the foods, recipes for the foods in the sirtfood diet, success stories, a meal plan, and answers to burning questions you might have. We have managed to go through all that and even more. The ball is in your court right now, and it is up to you to put the information that you have garnered from this book into good use. It is not too unusual for people to consume revolutionary information and not put them to good use. A lot of times, it takes just one book or one piece of information to change your life, and to be honest, this book could be your turning point. The sirtfood diet is so effective because its effects are noticed almost immediately, spurring you on to keep trying to make more progress. As has been described extensively in the book, the foods in the diet are packed with nutrients and biochemicals called polyphenols that would work in tandem with the calorie-restriction policy to help to activate a special set of genes in your body called the sirtuins. The sirtuins would then direct a series of biochemical reactions in your body, which would help to instigate the burning of accumulated fat deposits, enhance fitness and mental alertness, and reduce your susceptibility to chronic diseases in the long term. The foods that make up the sirtfood diet have also been shown to contain other extremely helpful biochemicals such as antioxidants that help to counteract the effects of free radicals on the body, thereby helping to slow down aging. The anticarcinogenic agents in most of the core sirtfoods help to reduce the risk of cancer. Most of the sirtfoods also contain antiinflammatory agents that help prevent inflammation in the long and short term. The sirtfoods are also loaded with a lot of nutrients, which help to boost the immune system, lower blood sugar, correct and manage bone defects and promote the long-term well-being of the human body. The possibilities that the sirtfood diet offers are practically endless. This is a fortuity for you to make a difference in your life by making a difference to work on what goes into your body. You want to be fit, trim, healthy, and mentally alert?

Lightning Source UK Ltd.
Milton Keynes UK
UKHW021302100521
383455UK00005B/49